Anti-inflammatory diet for beginners

The complete guide to reducing inflammation in our body, preventing or treating the resulting diseases and living a healthy life

GILLIAN WILLET

Table of Contents

Introduction

With so much pollution, tension and stress taking their toll on our health, the one thing that we can do to battle this is to have a nutrition rich anti inflammation diet.

Pollution causes free radical damage and also has serious inflammatory effects which have tremendous adverse effects on our health, leading to numerous ailments including psoriasis, cancer, auto immune diseases, Alzheimer's disease, heart diseases etc. Can an anti-inflammation diet help here?

Of course it can. In fact that is one of the best ways to come out victorious from this maze of diseases and disorders. An anti-inflammation diet should strictly consist of omega 3 fatty acids which have amazing anti-inflammatory properties. These fatty acids are essentially comprised of DHA (Docosahexanoic Acid) and EPA (Eicosapentaenoic Acid) fats.

Our body internally converts DHA into a substance called Resolvin D2 which is a potent and effective anti-inflammatory agent. It works by inhibiting the production of pro-inflammatory eicosanoids which reduce the inflammation significantly and provide instant relief from various ailments including the common ones like arthritis and gout.

If you want to make this beneficial fatty acid a part of your daily diet, one best and efficient way is to incorporate premium fish oil supplements in your health regimen. Make sure to choose the one having more DHA content than EPA.

This not only helps in ensuring the anti-inflammatory properties contained in DHA but also ensures ample supply of both DHA and EPA to the body. This is due to our body's ability to convert DHA into EPA as per its re□uirement.

Since the reverse reaction is difficult to attain, it is advisable to take a supplement containing more DHA content.

These supplements not only regularize and assure your receiving an anti-inflammation diet, it also ensures that you take it in optimal amounts. The good supplements have the optimal usage per serving specified on them which is one thing to be checked before choosing to incorporate them in your daily regimen.

This complete guide is fully packed with tons of information about both an anti-inflammation diet as well as how to incorporate it in your routine, I hope you are going to take it forward and put it to the test right away. Take the decision and take it soon, after all there is nothing better than enjoying good health for years to come.

Happy Reading.

Chapter 1

The Anti-Inflammatory Diet

Chronic inflammation is a type of inflammation that silently attacks the body causing disease and degeneration, and is also known as "silent inflammation". As the connection between silent inflammation and a host of diseases becomes clearer, the case for dietary and lifestyle changes that can combat inflammation has become stronger.

While it was always known that some conditions such as arthritis and acne were a result of acute inflammation in the body, there is mounting evidence that silent inflammation plays a role in heart disease, Alzheimer's, diabetes and some cancers, as well as in the ageing process. Chronic inflammation can be present undetected in your body for years, until it manifests in disease.

Silent inflammation has been linked with the buildup of cholesterol deposits in the arteries which can lead to heart disease. In a similar way, the risk of Alzheimer's disease increases with inflammation of brain tissue, as this results in the buildup of amyloid plaque deposits in the brain.

Having type 2 diabetes, or eating sugary foods contributes to silent inflammation in the body as a result of elevated blood sugar and insulin levels. Recent studies have also confirmed the link between inflammation and several types of cancers. Making the necessary lifestyle changes to fight inflammation, can protect you from its devastating effects.

There are molecules in the body called prostaglandins which play an important role in inflammation. It has been found that of the three main types of prostaglandins, two of them (PG-E1 and PG-E3) have an anti-inflammatory effect, while the third type (PG-E2) actually promotes inflammation. When there is an imbalance in the body between these prostaglandins, inflammation can result.

Prostaglandins are made in the body from essential fatty acids. You can assist your body in making anti-Inflammatory prostaglandins by eating vegetables, nuts, grains and seeds such as sesame and sunflower seeds.

On the other hand, foods that cause a spike in insulin levels, such as sugary foods, or foods with a high Glycemic load promote production of PG-E2 and increase inflammation.

A typical anti-inflammatory diet focuses on fighting inflammation through the consumption of foods that lower insulin levels.

To actively reduce inflammation, you should therefore eat foods that have a low Glycemic load, such as whole grains, vegetables and lentils, and consume healthy fats such as nuts, seeds, fish, extra virgin olive oil and fish. Spices such as turmeric, ginger, and hot peppers also reduce inflammation.

At the same time, you also need to reduce consumption of foods that are pro-inflammatory, such as red meat, egg yolks and shellfish.

Sugar is a key culprit in inflammation, and therefore you should also cut back on sugary foods. Inflammation can also be reduced by taking supplements such as fish oils which are high in Omega 3 fatty acids.

Chapter 2

The Benefits Of An Anti-Inflammatory Diet

People suffering from obesity have inflammation issues. Diabetes, arthritis and asthma are all associated with inflammation in the body. Not to mention the link to certain heart conditions and cancers.

Reducing the inflammation in your body with an anti-inflammation diet can cause an immediate change to how you feel, not to mention the long term effects of the dietary change on health and well-being.

The first step to adopting an anti-inflammatory diet is to understand the effects of foods on the body. Food provides nutrients and vitamins the body needs to survive. The idea of eating to live not living to eat is a huge push for the weight loss community, but this idea should not just be followed when needing to lose a few pounds.

Certain foods have high concentrations of anti-oxidants and natural anti-inflammatory nutrients that may reduce the effect of inflammation on the body. It is these foods that cornerstone the anti-inflammatory diet.

The Role of Omega 3 and Other Fatty Acids

Fatty acids are present in many foods that contain oil. The best natural source is fish like salmon and sardines. However, Omega 6 fatty acids are prevalent in western diets over Omega 3s. This is because common eaten foods like chicken, turkey, eggs, nuts and vegetable oils are rich in Omega 6 fatty acids.

What people don't realize, however, is that these fatty acids need to be balanced with Omega 3s for optimal health and anti-inflammatory action. Most western diets include 10 times more Omega 6s than Omega 3s. Some diets include as much as 30 times more. The optimal ratio is 4 parts Omega 6 to every 1 part Omega 3.

Increasing Omega 3 fatty acids in the diet can reduce inflammation in the body and thus reduce the effect of this condition on health and general well-being. Foods rich in Omega 3s include fish oil, kiwi, black raspberry and various nuts.

The most readily available source of Omega 3s is flaxseeds. Many people mistake fish oils for the best source, but flaxseed oils tend to have the most readily available Omega 3s that make absorption in the body easier. Flaxseed oils contain about 55% ALA (alpha-linoleic acid) which is an Omega 3 fatty acid.

Another simple change to reduce inflammation in the body is the reduction of fatty meats. Red meat is the worst of all meats for people suffering from inflammation. Choosing a leaner cut or a leaner alternative is a good option. Bison and venison are two options that tend to contain less fat.

Grass fed cows also have fewer inflammatory characteristics on the body. Fish, lean chicken, turkey, soybeans, tofu and soy milk are all lean choices for decreasing inflammation. But some of these meats tend to be higher in Omega 6s.

To combat the fatty acid imbalance that may be increasing inflammation, try cooking these meats in olive oil or adding flaxseed oil to the final dish to boost Omega 3s.

The Danger of Processed Foods

The worst food to eat when suffering from inflammation is a processed carbohydrate. These foods offer very little nutritional value and should be replaced with whole grain alternatives. All flour is wheat based, but processed flour is stripped of the healthy grain wholeness and bleached.

What are left are empty calories sure to swell the body even more. Simply replacing white bread with whole grain bread and white flour with whole wheat flour that is unbleached can make a big difference in how your body reacts to your diet.

Chapter 3

Eating Anti-Inflammatory Foods

Scientists have found that there is a relationship, in part, between what we eat and inflammation. They've even identified some compounds in food that can reduce inflammation and others that promote it.

There is still a lot to learn about just how diet and inflammation interact, and research, as of yet, is not at that point where a specific foods or groups of foods can be singled out as being beneficial for people with arthritis. We are beginning to get a clearer picture of how eating the right way can reduce inflammation.

So why are we so concerned about inflammation?

Inflammation is the body's natural defense to infections and injuries. When something goes wrong the body's immune system goes to work to inflame the area, which serves to get rid of the invader or to heal the wound. Inflammation can cause pain, swelling, redness, and warmth, but this goes away as soon as the problem is solved. This is good inflammation.

Then we have chronic inflammation, the type that's familiar to people with rheumatoid arthritis (RA), lupus, psoriatic arthritis, and other types of "inflammatory" arthritis. Chronic inflammation is the type that will not go away.

All the types of arthritis that are mentioned above are a disorder of the immune system creates inflammation and then doesn't know when to shut off. Inflammatory arthritis, chronic inflammation can have serious conse□uences, permanent disability and tissue damage can be one if it isn't treated properly. Inflammation has been linked to a full host of other medical conditions.

Inflammation has been found to contribute to atherosclerosis, which is when fat builds up on the lining of arteries, raising the risk of heart attacks. Also, high levels of inflammation proteins have been found in the blood of people with heart disease. Inflammation has also been linked to obesity, diabetes, asthma, depression, and even Alzheimer disease and cancer.

Scientists think that a constant level of inflammation in the body, even if the level is low, can have a number of negative effects. Research shows that diet can reduce inflammation; in theory an inflammation-lowering diet should have an effect on a wide range of health conditions.

Researchers have looked for clues in the eating habits of our early ancestors to discover which foods might benefit us the most. They believe those habits are more in tune to our eating habits with how the body processes and uses what we eat and drink.

Our ancestor's diet consisted of wild lean meats (venison or boar) and wild plants (green leafy vegetables, fruits, nuts, and berries). There were no cereal grains until the agriculture revolution (about 10,000 years ago).

There was very little dairy, and there were no processed or refined foods. Our diets are usually are high in meat, saturated (or bad) fats, and processed foods, and there is very little exercise. Nearly everything we eat is available close by or as far away as our computer and the click of a mouse.

Our diet and lifestyles are way out of whack with how our bodies are made from the inside out. While our genetic make-up has changed very little from our early beginnings, our diet and lifestyles have changed a great deal and the changes have gotten worse over the last 50 to 100 years.

Our genes haven't had a chance to adapt. We aren't giving our bodies the right kind of fuel, it's as though we think of our bodies as engines in a jet plane when instead they are like the engine in the very first planes.

There are some foods that we are putting into our bodies, especially because we are eating way too much of them, that are affecting our health in a bad way.

There are two nutrients in our diets that have attracted attention, are omega-3 fatty acids and omega-6 fatty acids have been part of our diets for thousands of years. They are components in just about all of our many cells and are important for normal growth and development.

Both of these acids play a role in inflammation. In several studies it was found that certain sources of omega 3's in particular, help to reduce the inflammation process and that omega 6's will raise it.

Now this is the problem, the average American eats on average about 15 times more omega 6's than omega 3's.

While our very early ancestor's ate omega 6's and omega 3's in equal ratio, and it is believed that this is what helped to balance their ability to turn inflammation on and off. The imbalance of omega 3's and omega 6's in our diets is believed to contribute to the excess of inflammation in our bodies.

So why is it that we eat so many omega 6's now? Vegetable oils such as corn oil, safflower oil, sunflower oil, cottonseed oil, soybean oil, and the products made from them, such as margarine, are loaded with omega 6's. Even many of the processed snack foods that are so readily available today are full of these oils.

Based on the best information of the time, was to use vegetable oils like those mentioned above instead of foods with saturated fats such as butter and lard. It looks like the conse☐uences of that advice may have contributed to the increased consumption of omega 6's and therefore causing an imbalance of omega 3's and omega 6's.

You can find omega 6's in other common foods such as meats and egg yolks. The omega 6 found in meat is the fatty acids that come from grain-fed animals such as cows, lambs, pigs and chickens.

Most of the meat sold in America is grain fed unlike their grass-fed cousins who contain less of those fatty acids. Wild game such as venison and boar are lower in omega 6's and fat and higher in omega 3's than the meat that comes from the supermarkets where we shop.

You can get omega 3s in both animal and plant food. Our bodies can convert omega 3s from animal sources into anti-inflammatory compounds more easily than the omega 3s from plant sources. Plant foods contain hundreds of other healthful compounds many of which that are anti-inflammatory, so don't discount them all together.

There are many foods that are high in omega 3s and that include fatty fish, especially fish from cold waters. Of course everyone knows about salmon but did you know that you can also find omega 3s in mackerel, anchovies, sardines, herring, striped bass, and bluefish.

It's also widely known that wild fish are better sources of omega 3s than the farm raised ones. You can also buy eggs that have been enriched with omega 3 oils. There are several excellent sources of omega 3s in plants that are leafy greens (like kale, Swiss chard, and spinach) as well as flaxseed, wheat germ, walnuts, and their oils.

You can also get omega 3s in supplements (often as fish oil); this source has been shown to be beneficial in some instances. You should take with your doctor before you take a fish oil supplement because it can interact with some medications and under certain circumstances can increase the risk of bleeding.

I take a prescribed omega 3 supplement because my doctor had told me that the ones you get in the supermarket or health food store are not pure, they have other additives that do absolutely nothing to help.

There are other fats that are contributors to clogged arteries, the "bad" or saturated fats found in meats and high-fat dairy foods, these are called pro-inflammatory.

There are also the Trans fats that are relatively new to the cause of heart disease. These Trans fats can be found in processed convenience and snack foods and can be spotted by reading the labels.

They can be identified as partially hydrogenated oils, often soybean oil or cottonseed oil. But, they can also occur naturally in small amounts in animal foods. The thought is that they contribute to the pro-inflammatory activities in our bodies and the amounts we eat today are staggering.

Antioxidants are substances that prevent inflammation causing "free radicals" from over taking our bodies. Plant foods such as fruits, vegetables (including beans), nuts, and seeds carry high amounts of antioxidants. Extra-virgin olive oil and walnut oil are very good sources of antioxidants, also.

These foods have long been considered the basics for good health, and can be found in fruits and vegetables with colorful and vibrant pigments.

The more colorful the plant, the better they are for you, from green vegetables, especially leafy ones, to low-starch vegetables, such as broccoli and cauliflower, to berries, tomatoes, and brightly colored orange and yellow fruits and vegetables.

We don't have to revert back completely to the caveman to eat the anti-inflammatory way to benefit from the anti-inflammatory diet. Just eating a healthful diet that is recommended today is right on track.

Our chief strategy should be to balance the amount of modern day foods with the foods of long ago, which were rich in the inflammation reducing foods.

Really, all we have to do is replace foods rich in omega 6 with foods rich in omega 3, cutting down on how much meat and poultry we eat while eating oily fish a couple of times a week and adding more varieties of colorful fruits and vegetables, and while whole grains were not a part of our early ancestor's diet, it should be included in ours.

Be sure that it is whole grains and not refined grains because they contain many beneficial nutrients and inflammation-tempering compounds. Researchers have found that eating a lot of foods high in sugar and white flour may promote inflammation, although there is more studying that needs to be done on the subject.

The amounts of knowledge we have on how the body works and how our ancestor's ate is helping to confirm the old adage: "You are what you eat." But, there is still more we need to learn before we can prescribe any one anti-inflammatory diet.

Our genetic makeup and the severity of our health condition will determine the benefits we get from an anti-inflammatory diet and unfortunately there is doubt that there will be one diet that fits us all.

Also, what we eat or don't eat is just a small part of the whole story. We are not as physically active as our ancestors and physical activity has its own anti-inflammatory effects. Our ancestors were also much leaner than we are and body fat is active tissue that can make inflammatory producing compounds.

Anti-inflammatory eating is a way of selecting foods that are more in tune with what the body actually needs. We can achieve a more balanced diet by going back to our roots.

Chapter 4
Biggest Struggles Of An Anti-Inflammatory Diet

Everyone wants to feel better and live in better health. One of the easiest ways to achieve that is by switching from a traditional western diet to an anti-inflammatory diet. Making the change is easy, but much like a diet plan, sticking with the food changes and watching what you eat can be difficult.

Fast food is a huge hindrance to the anti-inflammatory diet. Foods that are high in fat tend to increase inflammatory substances in the body for three to four hours after the meal.

If the same number of calories eaten in one fast food sitting were eaten as fresh fruits, vegetables and lean meats, this effect would not occur. Free radicals, cell killers that compound inflammation problems, can also be increased by 175% after eating fast food.

The Alternative - The best alternative to fast food is a replacement, anti-inflammatory diet. Take the Big Mac from McDonald's into consideration. This sandwich can be made from lean ground turkey and a whole grain bun.

The "special" sauce can be mixed up with lower carbohydrate ketchup, olive oil mayonnaise and sugar free relish. The result is a tasty alternative with a significantly lower fat count.

Red Meat, Milk and Your Inflammation

Science has long fought to connect red meat with certain forms of cancer. Little did they know the research would lead to a link between this common dinner protein and inflammation. Researchers believe the body reacts to certain chemical aspects of red meat and milk in a protective manner.

If the body believes these are foreign substances, the immune system will kick in and inflammation occurs. Imagine eating red meat once a day and drinking two or three glasses of milk. The body would live in a state of constant or chronic inflammation which could cause health problems over time.

The Alternative - Lean poultry, beef and fish are all part of a healthy diet. Beef is a great source of iron, so eliminating it is not a necessity. But, choosing the leanest of cuts is essential to good health. The best meats are lean proteins and beans.

Trans Fats and Your Inflammation

A hidden source of body inflammation is the trans fatty acid. While many people know a bit about this type of fat, few understand the effects on the body. Fast food, baked goods, prepackaged meals and margarine are often good sources of trans fat.

After entering the body, these fats can increase the risk of coronary artery disease, insulin resistance, diabetes and heart failure. Increased risk of stroke due to abnormally high lipid levels is also common.

While many foods will claim to be trans-fat free, that is not the entire truth. According to labeling guidelines, these foods can contain up to 0.5 grams of trans fats per serving and still mark the product as "trans fat free". These small amounts will add up over time if the diet is rich in processed foods, margarine and baked goods.

Natural fats like whole butter and olive oil have no trans fats. Choosing these in place of hydrogenated oils and margarine is a good first step.

When it comes to foods cooked in trans-fat, there is no choice but to eliminate these from the diet all together. Many people choose to adopt an anti-inflammatory diet by baking their own snacks and cooking "fast food" style meals at home.

Chapter 5

Anti-Inflammatory Foods To Add To Your Diet

Inflammation is the first sign when something harmful or irritating is affecting parts of our body. Every one's body has an immune system and inflammation is part of that.

Inflammation is also a localized physical condition that results as a reaction to an injury or infection, causing parts of the body to become swollen, reddened, painful and hot. Internal inflammation can happen due to eating of processed foods, fats and sugars.

High levels of inflammation can cause a number of health complications such as arthritis, joint pain, damage to blood vessels among others.

To combat this, it is important you eat foods that are anti-inflammatory. Such foods are readily available to add to your diet to curb inflammation. Here are some of the foods and suggestions to help and keep harmful inflammation at bay:

Whole Grains

When it comes to whole grains it is better you consume your grains as whole grains and not refined or pasta. Research has shown that whole grains contain a high amount of fibre which reduces the inflammatory marker in blood known as C-reactive protein.

Dark Leafy Greens

Dark leafy vegetables such as spinach and kale have high concentrations of vitamin E and minerals such as calcium and iron. Studies show that vitamin E helps in protecting your body from inflammatory molecules known as cytokines. Additionally, dark leafy greens have a high amount of disease fighting phytochemicals.

Fatty Fish

Oily fish such as salmon and tuna are foods that are anti-inflammatory as they contain high amounts of omega 3 fatty acids. The fatty acids are known to help joint inflammation, so make sure you get plenty of omega 3. Another important fact about omega 3 is you must get it in your food because the body cannot make it within its system.

Soy

Soybeans contain isoflavones compounds which help the negative effects of inflammation on joints. However, it is good you avoid heavily processed soy products as they may contain additives and preservatives. Instead, include soy milk and soy beans into your regular diet.

Nuts

Nuts such as almonds and walnuts are rich in vitamin E, calcium and fibre. All nuts are full of antioxidants which can help the body in repairing the damages caused by inflammation.

Berries

Berries are low in fat and calories but rich in antioxidants. Their anti-inflammatory anthocyanins compound in them has many good ⬚ualities. This helps to prevent you from developing arthritis.

Green Tea

Green tea as well has anti-inflammatory flavonoids; this reduces the onset of inflammation and minimizes the risk of certain cancers. It shouldn't be underestimated for many other health benefits. It can reactivate skin cells making skin appear brighter. Drink it regularly and use some honey as a sweetener instead of sugar.

Low Fat Dairy

Low fat dairy such as yogurt contains probiotics which can prevent inflammation. Additionally, dairy foods that are anti-inflammatory such as skim milk with high calcium and vitamin D are important for everyone since apart from having anti-inflammatory properties, they strengthen your bones also.

Ginger and Garlic

Ginger and garlic are foods that are anti-inflammatory. Both are known to lower body inflammation, control blood sugar levels and help your body in fighting certain infections. Selenium and sulphur in garlic is an essential compound for a healthy immune system. It is also one of the top anti-aging foods you can eat.

Turmeric and Sweet Potato

Turmeric has natural anti-inflammatory compounds called curcumin which is known to turn off NF-kappa B protein that triggers the process of inflammation. On the other hand, sweet potato is a good source of fibre, vitamin B 6, vitamin C, complex carbohydrates and better carotene.

Wine

It's common knowledge that drinking wine in moderation is a good cardiac-protective activity. A lesser known quality of grape-based or red wine is that it is composed of high concentration of anti-inflammatory properties. To get the same effects, you can also consume fresh grapes since the skin contains the same features.

Olive Oil

Omega-3 is not the only source of fatty acids. It can be found in abundance in olive oil. the best way to utilize this is to cook your vegetables in olive oil. Studies have indicated that compared to raw veggies, those that have been cooked in olive oil produced more anti-inflammatory properties.

All of these anti-inflammatory foods have been touted by experts as being the most comprehensive and effective diet available. While there are other diet plans which offer similar results, depending upon your own personal circumstances, any diet rich in protein, oils and fiber is beneficial.

Chapter 6

How The Anti-Inflammatory Diet Can Protect You From Disease

Inflammation is a good thing. It is the natural way your body responds to threats such as infections or wounds. We have all seen inflammation at work when we have pain and redness at an injury. We say it looks inflamed, and it literally is, because injury activates the inflammatory response.

When inflammation lasts for long periods of time, we call it chronic, and it can cause problems. Some common causes of chronic inflammation include allergies, autoimmune disease, periodontal disease, arthritis and other diseases that activate the immune system over time. Even obesity is inflammatory, because fat cells give off chemicals called cytokines that trigger inflammation.

Chronic inflammation causes damage to the endothelial lining of arteries, which can lead to atherosclerosis and heart disease. There is also evidence that it contributes to type 2 diabetes, Alzheimer's disease and a growing number of other chronic diseases that are common in modern, western societies.

The symptoms of inflammation vary with what is causing it. You may even have no symptoms at all, as in the case of obesity. Here are some examples of specific disease related symptoms:

• Arthritis, rheumatoid arthritis (joint pain, stiffness, swelling)

• Crohn's disease or ulcerative colitis (abdominal pain and cramping, fever, diarrhea)

• Psoriasis or eczema (redness)

• Allergies (respiratory symptoms, hives)

More subtle, early indicators of problems could include headaches, muscles aches, fatigue, muscle stiffness, nausea, vomiting, diarrhea or constipation, gas, abdominal discomfort and even emotional problems including depression.

These could be related to food sensitivities and intolerances. The most common food intolerances include dairy (lactose), wheat (gluten), yeast, soy, corn, eggs and even some artificial sweeteners.

You can find out if you have inflammation by having your C- reactive protein levels tested. The high sensitivity C-reactive protein, is the preferred indicator of chronic, low-grade inflammation.

If your C-reactive protein levels are high, you will first want to talk to your doctor to find out if there is an underlying infection, allergy, autoimmune disorder or other contributing disease. If not, your excess weight could be the cause and weight loss is your best line of defense. If you are a smoker, that could also be contributing to the problem.

Inflammation can also be influenced by the foods you eat. Research has shown that certain foods trigger inflammation and others suppress it.

Some of the foods that are pro-inflammatory include:

Animal fats (corn-fed beef, dark meat and skin of poultry, pork, duck

Hydrogenated fats (trans fat)

Fried foods (fried in saturated,hydrogenated or polyunsaturated fats)

Sweets (sugar, candy, cookies, cakes, ice cream, donuts, sweet drinks)

Refined grains (white bread, pasta, white rice)

Processed foods (chips, crackers, fries, cold cuts, hot dogs, canned meats)

Dairy products (especially full fat milk, cheese, sour cream, cream cheese, cream)

Some people may also need to avoid the nightshades (potatoes, tomatoes, eggplant, peppers)

Here are some of the best anti-inflammatory foods:

Fatty fish such as salmon, sardines, herring, trout and tuna (with omega 3 fatty acids)

Grass fed beef also contain some omega 3 fats (unlike corn-fed beef, mostly saturated fats)

Nuts and seeds (walnuts, flaxseed, almonds)

Monounsaturated fats (olive oil, canola oil, avocados), by replacing polyunsaturated fats

Turmeric (part of most curry dishes)

Ginger, used in Asian cuisine (also helps control nausea)

Whole grains (except wheat, barley and rye if you are gluten intolerant)

Foods that have high antioxidant levels also tend to reduce inflammation, possibly by reducing the damage that stimulates inflammation. Antioxidants are prolific in brightly and darkly colored fruits and vegetables.

Some of the best sources of antioxidants include:

Berries: blueberries, raspberries, blackberries, cranberries, strawberries, cherries,

Beans: Red beans, kidney beans, pinto and black beans

Herbs: oregano, basil, sage, marjoram, thyme, dill, garlic, dry mustard

Spices: cinnamon, cloves, cumin, turmeric, ginger

Nuts: pecans, walnuts, pistachios

Green tea is rich in both antioxidants and anti-inflammatory compounds

Coffee, cocoa (or dark chocolate) and red wine (but caffeine and alcohol are inflammatory)

Exotic fruits: acai, gogi, pomegranate, papaya, pineapple

Eating more of these anti-inflammatory and high antioxidant foods can help calm chronic inflammation and by doing so, reduce your risk for chronic diseases. Find ways to make these foods a part of your everyday diet and you will not only be protecting your body from disease, but you may find that some of your aches and pains improve.

Chapter 7

Who Should Eat The Anti-Inflammatory Diet?

Most chronic diseases are a result of a lifestyle of affluence that affords us the luxury of being able to eat the wrong foods in the wrong amounts at the wrong times. These food choices set in play a host of processes in your body that produce inflammation from a multitude of sources.

In addition, many of us are genetically programmed to produce excessive inflammation when exposed to common irritant sources such as smoke, chemicals and poor dietary choices. Some of us produce so much inflammation that we have autoimmune disorders such as lupus, multiple sclerosis, rheumatoid arthritis, psoriasis and colitis.

How exactly do poor food choices produce inflammation?

Packaged and highly processed foods as well as fast foods are some of the worst culprits. They are also some of the food choices most widely available. Designed for convenience, these foods are loaded with trans-fat to extend their shelf life as well as change their taste and texture.

A trans-fat is created from a natural, saturated fat - another less than healthy fat. That saturated fat is "transformed" into a trans-fat via a process called trans-hydrogenation.

This transformed fat is chemically different enough from a natural fat that, when incorporated into your body tissues, it creates a cascade of chemicals called cytokines. Cytokines are molecules responsible for producing inflammation throughout your body.

Foods that are loaded with refined sugars are also inflammatory. Cakes, cookies and doughnuts are examples of foods that are rapidly digested by your body, releasing large amounts of glucose. This glucose is rapidly absorbed by your body, causing a high blood glucose level. Your body in turn releases a surge of insulin to help normalize your blood glucose levels.

This surge of insulin combined with high blood glucose levels causes your body to release cytokines, inflammatory molecules, as well. Each surge of glucose actually signals your body to store fat. Guess what? Fat tissue becomes physiologically active and begins to release these same inflammatory molecules, cytokines, as well.

Refined grains - grains stripped of fiber and vital nutrients- also create inflammation. A whole grain is a molecule composed of large amounts of glucose linked together and encapsulated with a fiber coating. This fiber coating makes the digestion and release of glucose a slow and steady process.

When the outer fiber coating is stripped away to create a smooth and creamy texture, glucose molecules are readily available for rapid digestion and absorption into your body. This rapid surge of glucose into your system again is the trigger for the inflammatory cascade.

Certain grains have the ability to produce inflammation in certain individuals. Wheat, oats, barley and rye are all grains that contain significant amounts of a protein substance called gluten. Gluten makes foods, like bread, crunchy on the outside and soft on the inside.

Yet this same gluten is very inflammatory in individuals genetically challenged in digesting gluten. Symptoms can be as severe as pain, bloating, diarrhea and malnutrition or as mild as nausea or lack of energy. Eliminating these specific grains from your diet is often the key to controlling this type of inflammation.

Inflammation affects every person in the world at some point in their life. In western cultures, like the United States, a huge portion of the population is affected by inflammation every day.

Being overweight or obese is the most common inflammatory condition. It is this inflammatory response that could be the cause of some weight related conditions like diabetes.

When fat cells grow, they take up the free space around the organs. Blood flow can be constricted and the body often feels as though it needs to fight to function normally.

When the body feels threatened, inflammation occurs as a natural, healing response. Unfortunately, unlike the small cut that will heal in a few, short days. Obesity takes time to correct and the longer the body lives inflamed, the greater the risk of long term effects.

In the case of obesity, changing the diet by reducing calories will reduce body weight and thus reduce the inflammation in the body. This is the simplest benefit of an anti-inflammatory diet. However, people who are obese or overweight are not the only people who can benefit from an anti-inflammatory diet.

There are many illnesses and conditions caused by inflammation. These include asthma, arthritis, inflammatory bowel syndrome, pelvic inflammatory disease, endometriosis, diabetes, COPD, Psoriasis, Colitis, and Lupus - just to name a few. All-in-all, there are nearly 40 autoimmune conditions currently accepted by the medical community that are affected by inflammation.

The first step is to make dietary changes to reduce food based inflammation. Processed foods, fast foods and prepackaged foods can cause increased inflammation in the body.

Replacing these foods with lean meats, whole grains and healthy fats will make a tremendous different in how the body reacts to inflammation. In addition, if weight is a problem, reducing weight while changing to an anti-inflammatory diet can increase the benefits exponentially.

Changing to an anti-inflammatory diet does not have to be in reaction to a disease or illness. Prevention is the best choice and the anti-inflammatory diet can reduce the risk of contracting many of the listed illnesses.

When the body feels as though it needs to fight for survival, inflammation occurs, so offering healthy foods that have an inflammatory effect is a great choice for all people including those who are young, healthy and feel they do not need an anti-inflammatory diet.

Chapter 8

Foods Hurting Your Anti-Inflammatory Diet

You have chosen to take your life and your health back and eat an anti-inflammatory diet. Many people are making the same choice to fight the effects of obesity, diabetes, arthritis and other inflammatory conditions. As is the case with any dietary change, after a time, the control once assumed over the foods eaten can grown lax.

Often, the same foods will creep back into the diet and reduce the efficacy of the anti-inflammatory diet. These are packaged foods, oil blends and margarine. Reducing protein and water intake are the remaining common factors.

Packaged foods are just plain bad for the body. Often these foods contain enough sodium and dietary fat for an entire day. While it may seem harmless to pop a meal in the microwave two or three times a week, the impact can be dramatic.

On average, prepackaged meals have between 700 and 1000 calories each. Just three meals a week can contribute an additional 3000 calories to the diet, not to mention the increases in fat and sodium. High fat meals cause inflammation in the body for hours after consumption and can lead to weight gain which is causes more inflammation.

Oil blends are easier on the budget than pure olive oil. These blends, however, can include oils that contain trans fats. These fats are unhealthy and should not be consumed at ALL in the diet. Saving a bit of money on the front side may be counteracting your good anti-inflammatory diet choices on the back side.

Margarine is cheaper and contains fewer calories than butter. Some people even believe that eating pure butter can cause an increase in cholesterol levels which may lead to stroke. This is NOT the case.

People who choose to eat very low carbohydrate diets, which often include high butter intakes, measure lower cholesterol numbers than their margarine or low fat eating peers.

Protein is expensive and lean protein can break the budget. When money is tight, buying that fatty burger to replace the 93/7 lean beef that was part of your anti-inflammatory diet may seem like a harmless choice. Fatty red meat is linked to an increased risk of cancer and causes inflammation in the body. Instead, try replacing the burger, all together, will beans.

Water is the fluid of life and drinking water is the best choice for bettering overall health and decreasing inflammation. Many people start off an anti-inflammatory diet by drinking a half gallon of water a day or more.

Over time, lax behavior may lead to increased caffeine intake and reduced water intake. Caffeine is linked to inflammation and can cause the anti-inflammatory diet to work less effectively at reducing inflammation.

The anti-inflammatory diet is not about strictly forbidding all foods that may increase inflammation. Deprivation is the number one reason people scrap new diets and return to old eating habits. Instead of depriving, try healthier alternatives or simply reduce the number of times prepackaged foods, fatty red meats and trans fat based oils are eaten.

Chapter 9

Anti-Inflammatory Diet Plan

Inflammation triggers a response from the immune system. Initially inflammation is beneficial as it is used for protection but a lot of the time inflammation can lead to further inflammation (Chronic) which leads to big health problems.

There are certain foods contained in many people's diet today which lead to an increase in inflammation. You can probably guess what kinds of foods these are (fake foods, fried foods, processed foods, refined carbs, coffee, alcohol).

The anti-inflammatory diet contains many foods, which I have recommended for other purposes which help to stop and reduce inflammation. It is a very natural way of improving your health and recovering from illness or injury.

Without inflammation to worry about you will be a lot healthier and less at risk of picking up some very harmful illnesses in the long run.

Healthy fats make up a large proportion of the anti-inflammation diet. Foods high in Omega-3 fatty acids have been proven to be anti-inflammatory so I recommend eating as many of these foods to help fight inflammation.

Fish is a great source so stock up on sardines, salmon, herring and anchovies. Other good sources include extra virgin olive oil, coconut oil, avocado oil and walnuts.

Antioxidant Rich Fruit and Vegetables

Fruit and vegetables are packed full of antioxidants and vitamins, some of these vitamins are proven to be anti-inflammatory. Some of the best sources of vegetables include onions, spinach, sweet potato, peppers, garlic, broccoli and other green leafy vegetables.

Good fruits and berries to look out for are blueberries, papaya, pineapple and strawberries. They are packed with high antioxidant content which is great on such a diet.

High Quality Protein

Which proteins you eat are very important. There is a big difference between cheap value meats and grass fed organic meats. The cheap value meats will most likely be packed with hormones and pesticides, which lead to inflammation, whereas grass fed organic meat will help to fight inflammation.

Pick your meat wisely and go for the omega-3 packed grass fed versions as often as you can. Use this rule when it comes to eggs as well.

Steak, fish, eggs and poultry and beans (legumes).

These three types of foods form the cornerstone of the anti-inflammation diet.

Also herbs and spices including ginger, curcumin, turmeric, oregano and rosemary contain important substances which reduce inflammation and help to limit dangerous free radical production.

Food to Avoid at All Costs on an Anti-Inflammation Diet

I have just mentioned the foods that can lead to a reduction of inflammation which will keep you healthy. These foods I'm about to mention are the foods which cause inflammation and you should really avoid these.

So if you regularly eat any of the above foods just mentioned then you need to start to cut them out. Eating these types of foods on an anti-inflammation diet completely defeats the purpose of what you are trying to do and will ruin your results.

Even if you don't suffer from inflammation but want to change your eating habits then following this type of diet will still be good for you. It will increase your health greatly and will help with fat loss.

The next steps would be to begin to introduce anti inflammation foods into your diet. Begin with adding the healthy omega 3 fats. Start to use extra virgin olive oil with your vegetables, coconut oil with your cooking, start snacking with nuts instead of chocolate bars and crisps and start to eat more fresh fish. Supplementing with a high □uality fish oil supplement is also very important.

Chapter 10
Steps To Start Eating Healthier Today

There are many ways to stop the effect your diet has on inflammation. The easiest is adopting an anti-inflammation diet. Here are the three beginning steps to starting the diet off right.

Fruits, Vegetables and Seafood are good.

Vegetables that offer a deep color are often better for your health. These deep colors often mean higher fiber content and better anti-inflammatory effects on the body. Herbs are also fantastic additions to an anti-inflammation diet. Here is a list of foods and herbs that will best help you to gain control over your inflammation.

- Turmeric

- Oregano

- Garlic

- Green Tea

- Blueberries

- Ginger

- Wild Seafood

- Spinach

- Collard Greens

- Kale

When choosing seafood, the smaller the fish the better. Mercury is present in all fish and this is a compounding element. Eating the smaller fish like sardines, means eating from the lower end of the food chain with less mercury.

The idea is to boost healthy foods and eliminate unhealthy foods so for every good food you choose as part of your anti-inflammation diet, try taking out a processed food or fatty meat.

Increase Essential Fatty Acids (EFAs)

There is talk all over the Internet and in print about the power of EFAs. These fatty acids are present in nearly every food we eat, but the ratio of the different fatty acids is important as well as general consumption. Most people consume far more Omega 6s than Omega 3s and that can reduce the healthiness of even the best anti-inflammation diet.

Foods rich in Omega 3s include fish oil, olive oil, avocado, walnuts and grapeseed oil. An Omega 3 supplement can also be taken to boost this EFA in the diet. While flaxseed oil is the best source of Omega 3s, a fish oil supplement can also be chosen. It is important to make sure the fish oil is mercury free and tested for heavy metals.

Nuts and seeds are also perfect sources of EFAs. There is nothing hard about adding a handful of nuts or seeds to a salad or as a snack every day. For people with nut allergies, soy provides a healthy alternative. Soy is also a good source of lean protein which also has an anti-inflammation effect.

You may also hear about Omega 9 fatty acids. These are naturally occurring in the body, but that does not mean the amounts of this EFA when compared to Omega 3 and Omega 6 should not be taken into consideration. The effect of EFAs is heavily dependent on balance.

So far, stepping into an anti-inflammation diet has been really easy. During the elimination phase, however, some people have trouble giving up the foods they have grown to love the most. When listing the foods that need to be eliminated for their inflammatory effect on the body in order of importance, the list would include:

• Trans Fats

• Sugar

• Refined Carbohydrates

• Potential Food Allergens

Trans fats are present in hydrogenated oils like margarine. Despite many labels ready "0 trans fats"; they are still in those products in small amounts. Sugar is just not good for the body.

Replacing processed sugar with natural cane may be a healthier alternative. Refined carbohydrates include processed flour which is used in nearly every loaf of bread and baked goods sold in a package. Try baking for yourself with whole grain flour instead.

Food allergens often include gluten, soy, eggs, dairy and nuts. These foods will increase inflammation in the body immediately if there is a food allergy.

Medical food allergy testing can provide a specific list of food that will cause a reaction in the body. If you want to find out which foods you are allergic to on your own, keep a journal and eliminate the foods one by one for a few days.

Then, eat the food in question to see if there is a change or reaction. Mild food allergies often affect gastrointestinal systems with constipation or diarrhea. Rashes and hives, both inflammatory responses, may also appear.

Chapter 11

How To Cure Sciatica With An Anti-Inflammatory Diet

Increased consumption of processed foods has led directly to an increase in pain and discomfort related to inflammation in the body, including sciatica. Sciatica occurs when inflammation puts pressure on the sciatic nerve, causing pain in the lower back and down one or both legs. Foods rich non-inflammatory ☐ualities are one answer for how to cure sciatica at home.

Inflammation is the body's natural reaction to injury or infection. It can be beneficial when the systems of the body are working to repair themselves. However, modern diets have led to an abundance of inflammation without a purpose, which poses a variety of problems.

Many people use NSAIDs, or anti-inflammatory medications such as ibuprofen, to relieve pain from inflammation. However, most do not consider the risks of NSAID overuse.

The most common issue that arises from using anti-inflammatory drugs is gastrointestinal pain. In serious cases, long-term NSAID users experience fatal ulcers and other life-threatening ailments. An anti-inflammatory diet is an alternative to medication.

How to Cure Sciatica at Home with an Anti-inflammatory Diet:

1. Eat anti-inflammatory foods. Kelp, Wild Alaskan Salmon, Turmeric, Shitake Mushrooms, Papaya, Blueberries, Broccoli, and Sweet Potatoes are some popular anti-inflammatory foods. Not only will these foods help reduce swelling, thereby, decreasing pain, they will also provide balanced nutrition and taste great.

2. Drink anti-inflammatory drinks. Drinking plenty of water and green tea will reduce swelling, redness, and discomfort associated with inflammation. Adults should drink 8 glasses of water per day.

Water will have the added benefits of reducing appetite and clearing skin. In addition to reducing inflammation, green tea has also been shown to decrease the risks of cancer and heart disease.

3. Cook with Extra Virgin Olive Oil. EVOO is the Mediterranean secret to good health. The abundant supply of polyphenols is vital in reducing inflammation in the heart and blood vessels. The monounsaturated fats in olive oil are used by the body as anti-inflammatory agents, decreasing asthma and rheumatoid arthritis.

4. Supplement fish oils. If you are not eating 2 portions of oily fish per week, use fish oil

supplements to decrease inflammation. You are looking for 2-3 grams a day of EPA and DHA. Ginger and turmeric supplements are also very beneficial to your health.

If you have been experiencing chronic pain, try an anti-inflammatory diet before use of risky medications or invasive surgeries. If you have been looking for an answer for how to cure sciatica at home, start with sensible food choices.

Additionally, you should try increasing the amount of exercise you are doing regularly. Walking and stretching are ideal ways to relieve pain.

Chapter 12

The Anti-Inflammatory Diet For Arthritis Relief

Food and arthritis have a connection to each other and that is why changing your diet is one of the first pieces of advice an expert can give a person with inflammation in his or her joints. There are foods that can reduce inflammation and there are those that might worsen the inflammation.

A person with arthritis should follow the anti-inflammatory diet if he or she wants to get treated. To start an anti-inflammatory diet, one should know which foods he or she going to eliminate in one's diet and which foods will be added.

What are the foods that you should avoid and eliminate in your diet? When it comes to arthritis, it is always advised that the person affected should eliminate artificial foods like junk foods, those foods that have been processed and foods with added artificial flavorings and colorings.

A person with arthritis should also avoid meats that have high levels of fats and foods that are high in sugar. The reasons why these kinds of foods should be avoided by people with arthritis is that the saturated fats and trans fats found in these kinds of foods can worsen one's condition.

He or she should also avoid potatoes, eggplants and tomatoes because these are part of the nightshade family of plant that contains solanine that can provoke the pain.

Cutting these kinds of vegetables in people with arthritis have not been proven yet to be effective, but those who followed this kind of diet often show improvements with their condition and find relief from pain.

What are the foods to be added in your diet if you have arthritis? If you already know which kinds of foods you should eliminate in your anti-inflammatory diet, you should now know foods to add to your diet:

1. Healthy fats and Oils: Fish oils are high in Omega-3 fatty acids that are essential to our health. This will help reduce the inflammation and prevent it from coming back. You will also get these fats in some seeds like flaxseed, pumpkin seeds, and sunflower seeds and also in Brazil nuts, almonds, cashew nuts and many more.

2. Fruits and Vegetables: You should be eating more fruits and vegetables if you have arthritis because these have a lot of mineral, vitamins, antioxidants and photochemical that are

beneficial for your arthritis and also to other conditions.

3. Protein: Eating more proteins like fishes and other seafoods and poultry meats will also help people with arthritis.

4. Drinks: You should need more liquids to keep your joints lubricated. Drink more water, fruit juices, tea, vegetable juice with low sodium and non-fat milk.

Chapter 13

Anti-Inflammatory Diet For Treating Our Nail Fungus

The anti-inflammatory diet can help boost your immune system, which can help fight off fungal infections. Drinking the recommended six to eight glasses of water a day is suggested with this diet, which can help to cleanse your inner system, also helping to fight off infection.

In addition to being helpful in the fight to rid oneself of a fungus infection, there are other health benefits attached to the diet such as help with depression and improved mental state, a stronger immune system, less water retainage and more.

The anti-inflammatory diet usually consists of eating 2,000 to 3,000 calories a day. The amount of calories depends on your size. You should be eating 40 to 50% of carbohydrates, 30 % of fat and include carbohydrates, fat and protein with each meal.

This diet uses a lot of fish and fresh fruits and vegetables while minimizing the consumption of fast food meals. Beans, winter s□uashes and sweet potatoes are also a big part of this diet. This diet is not typically meant for weight loss, but can be used for health reasons and is said to help with fungal problems.

It may take a little while for the diet to work. Remember, if you've been eating a totally different diet, particularly if it was a poor diet, it will take a while for your system to be completely cleaned out. You might want to make a visit to a nutritionist or to the local health food store to discuss how and when the diet will work.

You can expect any treatment to take six to twelve weeks to work and the change in your diet alone may not be enough. Keep a journal of what you eat and do and any changes you see if you are unsure of the effectiveness of treatment.

Again, this is something to be discussed with your healthcare physician, a dietitian or nutritionist or even your health foot store representative who is well-versed in dietary needs.

At times, a health foot store may have different or more reliable information than the internet or even your physician's office and may be able to give you some supplements, topical creams or organic lacquers which may prove to be extremely effective, especially in conjunction with the anti-inflammatory diet.

Chapter 14

How To Lose Weight And Feel Great With The Anti-Inflammatory Diet

The anti-inflammatory diet can make you feel great. "How," you ask. By cutting out or significantly reducing your consumption of pro-inflammatory foods. When these foods are cut from your diet, inflammation in the body reduces taking stress and strain from the joints and organs.

While following this diet your chance of weight loss also goes up. "How does this happen," by reducing your consumption of grain and wheat products, sodas, and other simple sugars that cause excess weight.

In short summary, the fewer inflammatory foods we eat, the less inflammation we have in the body.

Background Information on Pro-Inflammatory Foods:

Grains, refined sugars, partial-hydrogenated oils, vegetable and seed oils are from modern man. These foods have been around a short time; hence, obesity and disease are on the rise. Humans are genetically adapted to eat fruits, veggies, nuts, lean meats, and fish, foods not related to chronic diseases.

Why Do Grains Inflame?

Grains contain a protein called gluten. Gluten is the main cause of many digestive diseases, such as celiac disease, also contributor to frequent headaches.

They also have a sugar protein called lectins which has been shown to cause inflammation in the digestive system. Grains also contain phytic acid which is known to reduce the body's absorption of calcium, magnesium, iron, and zinc.

Lastly, grains contain high amounts of fatty acid biochemicals called omega-6 fatty acids which do cause inflammation. Fatty acid biochemicals known as omega-3 fatty acids are anti-inflammatory and found in fresh fish and green vegetables.

What Should I Eat?

Anti-inflammatory foods

All fruits and vegetables (raw or lightly cooked)

Red and sweet potatoes

Anti-inflammatory omega-3 eggs

Raw nuts

Spices such as ginger, turmeric, garlic

Organic butter, coconut oil, extra virgin olive oil

Fresh fish, avoid farm raised

Meat, chicken, eggs from grass-fed animals

Wild game such as deer, elk, etc.

Water, organic green tea, red wine, stout beer

Chapter 15

Anti-Inflammatory Diet To Slow Down Cellular Aging

Chemical oxidation of cells is a natural process for the body. However, these have some bad effects to the DNA and to electrons. When the cells undergo energy conversion process, the body produces harmful free radicals.

These free radicals are single electrons that follow a unique path. When they meet paired electrons in your system, they snatch one of the paired electrons. This leads to cellular inflammation and DNA damage.

Cellular inflammation plays a huge role in the accelerated process of skin aging. Wrinkles appear faster and skin tissues become more fragile. Eventually, this leads to the loss of dermis elasticity. Thin skin condition and saggy dermis are just some of the problems you might have to deal with in the future.

One of the best ways to prevent cellular aging is to have an anti-inflammatory diet. Basically, foods rich in antioxidants are consumed. Antioxidants are molecules that fight harmful free radicals. These molecules also prevent the formation of free radicals.

Here are some tips on how to slow down cellular aging:

1. Instead of eating junk foods for your snack, eat dark colored berries instead. Blackberries, blueberries and raspberries contain a hefty amount of antioxidants that can fight cellular aging. In addition to that, they are also rich sources of vitamins and minerals that can help fight the over-all skin aging process.

2. Always have vegetable side dishes for your main meals. Green leafy vegetables are rich

sources of antioxidative molecules. They can further avoid cellular aging.

3. Increase your intake of cold water fish like Tuna and Salmon. They are the best sources of omega-3 fatty acids DHA and EPA. According to experts, nothing can prevent cellular inflammation more than omega-3 fatty acids. These fatty acids prevent inflammatory problems of any kind. This can even reduce joint inflammation so you can have better health.

A good diet is fundamental to young looking skin. But in addition to that, you also need to feed your skin with a natural moisturizer that contains beneficial ingredients like CynergyTK, Phytessence Wakame and Nano Lipobelle HEQ10.

CynergyTK is an ingredient found in the wool of sheep. This ingredient is made up of functional keratin, a complex type of protein needed for the production of collagen. Phytessence Wakame is a type of sea kelp that can prevent the sudden loss of hyaluronic acid.

This acid is essential for collagen lubrication. Nano Lipobelle HEQ10 is an antioxidant that can further avoid cellular inflammation. This has smaller molecular properties so it can easily penetrate the skin.

Chapter 16

How To Beat Inflammation Naturally

Most people who experience inflammation have heard all about the medications that are available to cure the pain and swelling that can occur during a flare up.

But how many know that there are some great anti-inflammatory foods that can affect how you feel and reduce the pain associated with inflammation. Following an anti-inflammatory diet will help you beat inflammation naturally.

Inflammation is a swelling that may cause pain, discoloration and even the loss of movement. Usually most people experience severe inflammation when they are the sufferers of arthritis and when they have problems like heart disease and strokes.

Usually your doctor will recommend that you get sleep and exercise in moderation. He may also suggest lowering your weight and taking steroid based drugs or undergoing joint replacement surgery.

The medications do work fairly well in reducing the inflammation but often come with some serious side effects, such as ulcers and kidney problems. This may make you wonder if they are worth taking and whether using them is trading one illness for another.

Just like there are some foods that decrease inflammation, there are some that will increase the likelihood that you will get inflammation. These foods are junk foods, fast foods, sugar, and fatty meats.

Processed foods that contain Trans and saturated fats also increase the risk of inflammation. Other large contributors of saturated fats are dairy products and eggs.

By simply choosing low fat milk, low fat cheese and leaner cuts of meat, you can lower the risks of inflammation, as well as cut down on the chances of chronic disease and obesity. Other foods that increase inflammation include presweetened cereals and soft drinks.

In addition to these, there are foods that are high in sugar and foods that come from the plants labeled as nightshade type. These add to the risk of discomfort associated with inflammation.

Eating whole fruits and vegetables will give you the natural healing factors. However, not all vegetables work that way. Potatoes, eggplant and tomatoes can actually make inflammation worse.

In general, eat an abundance of fresh vegetables and fruits, whole grains, anti-inflammatory fats and nuts while limiting processed foods, meat protein, milk products, refined sugars, artificial colors/flavors/sweeteners and food sensitivities.

Vegetables:

Eat and Enjoy:

Enjoy an abundance of fresh vegetables and fruits in a variety of colors (preferably organic). Fruits and vegetables are full of vitamins, minerals, antioxidants and fiber which give the body the essential building blocks for health.

Examples include beans, squash, lintels, sweet potatoes, cruciferous vegetables, avocados, dark leafy greens... There are so many choices. As for fruits, pineapple and papaya are particularly good because they are high in bromelain, a powerful natural anti-inflammatory. Fruits and vegetables also make great, healthy snacks.

Avoid / Limit:

Avoid produce that is not grown organically. Toxic chemical residues from herbicides and pesticides can remain and when ingested are foreign irritants to the system. Many crops in North America are also genetically engineered and are put on the market without rigorous scientific study to determine safety for human consumption.

Independent research is finally being done to show toxic effects of consuming genetically modified organisms (2). Foreign DNA is randomly inserted into the genome of a crop. Examples include herbicide resistant corn and soy which are resistant to the herbicide Roundup, made by Monsanto. Roughly 90% of all corn and soy sold in North America is genetically modified.

Also be aware of derivatives of genetically modified ingredients (such as corn starch and corn syrup etc.). It has also been suggested that consuming GMOs is a contributing factor to the rise in allergies as our bodies are recognizing these food substances as foreign (3). By choosing items with the "certified organic" label, you avoid both GMOs and toxic herbicides/pesticides.

For some people, vegetables in the nightshade family may pose a concern. Examples of nightshade vegetables include tomatoes, peppers, potatoes and eggplant.

Nightshades contain alkaloids which are thought to exacerbate inflammation and joint damage in certain susceptible individuals with arthritis (though research is conflicting). Thus, for some individuals, limiting or avoiding nightshade vegetables may be beneficial.

Fats:

Eat and Enjoy:

Enjoy healthy, anti-inflammatory fats including olive oil, coconut oil, avocados, nuts, salmon and sardines. In humans, there are two essential fatty acids, alpha-linolenic acid (an omega-3) and linoleic acid (an omega-6). These are "essential" because they are required for good health but the body does not synthesize them. Omega-3 fats are anti-inflammatory.

Omega-6 fats can be pro-inflammatory or anti-inflammatory (as it can be metabolized by two different pathways). Researchers suggest that keeping the ratio of omega-6 to omega-3 between 2:1 and 4:1 is best for health.

The modern diet tends to be high in omega-6 as it is abundantly available in cooking oils. Thus, including rich sources of omega-3 is important (such as fish, flax and walnuts especially).

Avoid / Limit:

Fats to limit or avoid include margarine, butter, shortening, hydrogenated oils, trans fats, saturated fats, and milk fat. Omega-6 fats are very high in corn oil, safflower oil and sunflower oil. Trans fats are linked with inflammatory diseases (4).

Meat:

Eat and Enjoy:

In general, limit animal proteins because they tend to acidify the body and also promote inflammation. When selecting animal protein, enjoy fish, poultry (especially free-range and organically raised), lamb and omega-3 eggs.

Avoid / Limit:

Limit beef, pork, shellfish and factory farmed eggs. In general, grass-fed is superior to grain-fed. Avoid charred foods, smoked foods and cold cuts. Cold cuts contain nitrates and nitrites which promote cancer. Barbequed foods contain polycyclic aromatic hydrocarbons (PAHs) and heterocyclic amines (HCAs) which also promote cancer.

Dairy:

Eat and Enjoy:

Enjoy dairy substitutes in moderation (such as almond milk).

Avoid / Limit:

Avoid or limit dairy products in general. This includes milk, yogurt, cheese and ice cream. As we age, we lose the enzyme that digests dairy, resulting in lactose intolerance and inflammation. The milk protein, casein, is also acidifying which (despite what many people are brought up thinking) robs the bones of calcium.

Grains:

Eat and Enjoy:

Enjoy whole grains as opposed to refined grains. Refined grains are grains in which the germ and bran have been removed. This means there is loss of fiber, minerals and vitamins. In other words, the good stuff is removed in exchange for a longer shelf life. Some good examples of healthy grains include (organic) whole wheat/oats/bulgar/coucous, quinoa and whole oats (like steel-cut oats).

Whole grains are also a rich source of complex carbohydrates. Complex carbohydrates (as opposed to simple sugars) will prevent spikes in your blood sugar level. Sugar promotes inflammation.

Avoid / Limit:

Avoid or limit refined carbohydrates such as white bread, pastries, sweet things and pastas.

Nuts:

Eat and Enjoy:

Enjoy nuts and nut butters such as almonds, walnuts, sesame seeds, pumpkin seeds and flax.

Avoid / Limit:

Avoid any specific nut allergies.

Beverages:

Eat and Enjoy:

Enjoy plenty of pure, filtered water (avoiding chlorine, fluoride and other contaminants which are irritants that promote inflammation). Other great choices are lemon water and herbal teas.

Avoid / Limit:

Avoid sugary sodas, fruit juice (with sugar added) and milk.

Spices:

Eat and Enjoy:

Many spices reduce inflammation. Some great examples are turmeric, oregano, rosemary, ginger, garlic and cinnamon. Bioflavenoids and polyphenols reduce inflammation and fight free radicals. Cayenne pepper is also anti-inflammatory, as it contains capsicum. Capsicum is often used in pain-relief creams.

Sweeteners:

Eat and Enjoy:

Enjoy stevia, molasses, maple syrup or honey as better alternatives for refined sugar.

Avoid / Limit:

Avoid refined sugar, fructose and especially high fructose corn syrup which promote inflammation. Avoid artificial sweeteners.

Other:

Eat and Enjoy:

Enjoy fermented foods such as kimchi, miso soup and sauerkraut. Fermented foods are probiotic and help to rebuild the immune system by supporting healthy microflora in the gut and to reduce inflammation. Fermented foods also tend to be easy to digest and are also factories for B vitamins.

Avoid / Limit:

In general, eliminate processed foods, artificial colors, artificial flavors and preservatives. Also avoid foods that you have a known sensitivity or allergy to as this promotes inflammation.

Low grade sensitivities are easy to miss, so if you're unsure, have a food allergy test. Some of the most common problem foods include wheat (gluten), corn, soy, milk and nuts.

Chapter 17

Anti-Inflammatory Herbs And Natural Sources

The concept of anti-inflammatory herbs is s very interesting one in the world of naturopathy and natural health. The reason why I gravitate towards them is because in the realm of inflammation and anti-inflammatory diets, they're a nice middle ground. Some people call for a total anti-inflammatory diet, eating only foods that promote the quelling of inflammation in the body.

Others are on the Standard American Diet, eating a host of foods that are known to cause inflammation in the body and aggravate many disorders and conditions. Anti-inflammatory herbs are a nice in-between. Foods in general are said to be either pro inflammatory or anti-inflammatory.

As you might have guessed, foods that are pro inflammatory will increase the amount of inflammation occurring in different parts of your body, will increase the pain associated with it, and may also increase your risk of having chronic disease. Foods pro inflammatory are most junk foods, sugars, fast foods, highly processed foods, and meats high in fat.

But that seems a bit excessive. That's why I love the idea of anti-inflammatory herbs. They're a nice middle ground in the world of inflammation, allowing you to stay healthy in that arena without putting too much of a focus on inflammation in general.

Regularly eating some form of natural anti-inflammatory foods is key because it helps reduce the risk of things like arthritis and chronic autoimmune diseases. And due to the fact that herbal concoctions are generally fairly strong, anti-inflammatory herbs are a great addition to meals, as well as in supplements.

Herbs generally have a wide variety of health benefits, and because inflammation is a somewhat complex process in the body, herbs can affect inflammation in different ways. Inflammation, when carried beyond reasonable limits, can become a type of autoimmune condition.

It begins as negative stimuli causes white blood cells to activate in order to protect the area being negatively affected. Inflammation is necessary to the healing process, but chronic inflammation can cause lots of long term problems and is often excessive, like an allergic reaction.

Here are some of the best, most powerful anti-inflammatory herbs:

1. Turmeric. Turmeric is a spice very common to most Indian foods. Though it has many other medicinal benefits, turmeric is a powerful anti-inflammatory herbs. But it takes a bit of time to start working, so if you don't like the taste of turmeric, you might want to think about taking it in capsule form.

2. Ginger. Ginger is also a spice that is used very often in Asian cooking. This spice also has a potent flavor and takes a bit of time in order to take effect within the body.

Ginger is very versatile, being used in a range of both foods and drinks, so filling your diet with it shouldn't be too much of a challenge. You can drink ginger tea, ginger ale, use ginger in baked goods and spice meats with it.

3. Omega 3 Essential Fatty Acids. Though these aren't technically herbs, omega 3 essential fatty acids are something that everyone needs more of in their diets. They're not only anti-inflammatory, they have a range of other medicinal benefits all across the body.

4. Licorice. Licorice is another herb that is very effective in the world of anti-inflammation. This too is a great herb to take because of its diversity. Licorice is nice because it can be added to just about anything, like candy, tea, baked goods, vegetables, meats, and more, making it easy to get a high daily dose.

5. Mangosteen Juice. Mangosteen is a fruit native to Asia that has very powerful anti-inflammatory properties. Mangosteen juice is becoming more and more popular with persons who are suffering from the pain of arthritis, and mangosteen even has a very nice flavor. Many

people substitute it for orange juice in their morning breakfast.

A few others worthy of note are:

- Pineapple juice

- Chamomile

- Black Seed Oil

- White Willow

- Red and Black Pepper

- St John's Wort

- Cilantro

- Cinnamon

- Garlic

- Cloves

Chapter 18
Omega-3 Anti-Inflammatory Supplements

An omega-3 anti-inflammatory supplement is a natural nutritional supplement that has omega-3 fatty acids as its nutrient and benefits source, which is significant because omega-3 has very strong properties from being able to reduce and also inhibit inflammation.

Taking a supplement to manage inflammation is very beneficial because of the importance in keeping excess inflammation from building up in your body and becoming a chronic condition.

If this happens you will largely increase your risks for many different serious health problems, including an increased risk of heart disease and dying from a heart attack.

Additionally, joint problems and arthritis are a common condition, with millions of people suffering from their symptoms, and would very much benefit from an omega-3 anti-inflammatory supplement.

Where Does Omega-3 Come From?

Omega-3 is found in many plants and animals, but there are a few things that are significant to note:

(1) Omega-3 are essential fatty acids, meaning that people need them but they are not made by our bodies, so the must be ingested through diet or supplements.

(2) Omega-3 is not a single fatty acid but a group of fatty acids.

(3) All omega-3 fatty acids do not have the same anti-inflammatory properties.

Keeping these things in mind, the omega-3 fatty acids that have the strongest anti-inflammatory benefits come from omega-3 DHA, with fish oil from cold water fish and green lipped mussels probably being the 2 best sources. On the other hand omega-3 ALA, which is found in plants like flax, does not have inflammation reducing properties.

You especially hear about fish oil omega-3 supplements related to heart health. These are recommended by many heart health professionals, and the American Heart Association strongly recommends for people to increase the amount of fish in their diets - although this would be healthy and a good idea, getting the fish oil from a supplement will give a higher concentration source and further maximize the benefits.

For those with joint problems and arthritis, the green lipped mussel supplement omega-3 is likely more effective.

Like the fish oil, the green lipped mussel will be a very good source for the omega-3 DHA anti-inflammatory, but the mussel supplements will also include omega-3 ETA. This fatty acid is a COX-2 inhibitor, which will help inhibit or keep inflammation from returning to your joints after it is reduced or eliminated.

So, when you start an omega-3 anti-inflammatory supplement, you will want to look at green lipped mussel supplements or fish oil supplements, with part of the decision being related to the specific reason for wanting a supplement to get rid of inflammation - but actually, if you will take both of these together you will receive synergistic benefits, and have the most effective anti-inflammatory alternative.

Chapter 19

Natural Anti Inflammatory Foods For Better Health And Less Pain

Inflammation is recognized by pain, swelling, redness and heat around the affected area. There are different options to treat inflammation. One is medicines, which so far hasn't been most successful because it doesn't really cure the problem.

The other option is the natural way, from where our body originates from; our body been made by nature and gets its natural products from nature.

This means selecting the food that your body needs, because shortfalls of some ingredients most likely caused the illness in the first place. It is also understood our body can react different to foods, because some foods being metabolized different to others.

What that means, as in inflammation some foods can have a positive or a negative result. Here are some of the natural anti-inflammatory foods; if selected correctly they will make that difference in healing.

Natural Anti Inflammatory Foods

Vegetables and fruits: Vegetables and fruits of green and bright colour help the process of inflammatory conditions. Vegetables and fruits are rich in antioxidants such as vitamins, minerals, fibre which the body needs every day to stay healthy.

There are many varieties, per example, squash, sweet potatoes, avocados, beans, lentils, dark green leafy vegetables and cruciferous vegetables. All of these have many antioxidants, phytochemicals and anti-inflammatory properties present.

Important Fats

Also rich in anti-inflammatory foods are olive oil, coconut oil, salmon, sardines, and avocados. All of them contain omega 3 fatty acids which are essential for inflammation and joint health. The acid from omega 3 is an inflammatory agent that changes into prostaglandins which is a hormone like substance.

Omega 3 is not only beneficial for joint pain and inflammation, it is also important for health in general. We only can get omega from our diet, therefore it is important to include some of the healthy oils such olive, coconut, macadamia and krill, which is stronger than fish oil. There are many options of foods available which contain a variety of omega.

Oils you should know about

Olive oil has more health benefits than most people realise. Make sure to use it in your diet as much as possible. Olive oil is high in antioxidants and is containing a substance called oleuropein. Medical science has determined that extra virgin olive oil is one of the healthiest foods we can add to our diet.

This oil is most helpful and effective for arthritis sufferers because it can cool inflammation and ease joint pain. However, for cooking, frying, baking etc. use only coconut or macadamia nut oil.

Other oils when heated become toxic and usually turn into trans fats which can trigger inflammation and joint pain, as well as other health issues. Avoid these oils: Vegetable oils, soy bean, canola, these are the more common ones most people know about because of the names. Yes, they have a healthy sounding name, but they are not healthy.

Spices

Turmeric would be on top of the list in reducing inflammation and joint pain. As well turmeric has a compound curcumin which is known for many health benefits and has the power to cure joint pain. It is best used in its natural powdery form and added to your diet when possible, the more the better.

Other important spices used for reducing inflammation are cinnamon, rosemary, garlic, ginger and oregano. These are high in polyphenols and bioflavonoids which help to reduce inflammation as well as fight off free radicals. Cayenne pepper is also known for its anti-inflammatory property and its capsicum content which is added to some creams for pain relief.

Grain

Whole grains which contain carbohydrates can also help in preventing spikes in the sugar level of the blood, as it is known that sugar promotes inflammation.

However, use only non-refined whole grains, once processing has taken place all the goodness is lost, such as vitamins, minerals and fibre. Among the best grains are oats: Whole oats, whole wheat, quinoa, couscous and Bulgar.

To take a multi supplement is of benefit, it can fill the spot of some foods you otherwise may not get from your diet as needed daily. However, your first priority must always be the diet, only than when taking a supplement you will get best value.

The right type of food and supplementation is crucial to treat arthritis, inflammation and joint pain. Multi vitamins that contain vitamin C, E, zinc, B 6, copper and boron are good to have included in your diet.

It has been found that some nutrients deficiency in patients could be the cause of suffering from arthritis. There is also strong evidence that exercise is just as important as your diet.

Anyone suffering with arthritis pain, the last thing you would think about is exercise. You avoid moving as little as possible because every time you move it creates pain.

In fact, exercise is the alternative to joint pain relief, because it breaks the tendency to favour your joints and to avoid movement. Avoidance of movement and exercise will ultimately make the pain worse and weakens the body.

Chapter 20

Tips For Practicing The Anti-Inflammatory Diet

Inflammation and aging go hand in hand as inflammation markers - especially the ESR (erythrocyte sedimentation rate) - slowly increase with each decade.

Many age-related diseases have inflammation as their common denominator and this is partially modulated by diet, so here are 10 easy tips to avoid the buildup of damaging inflammation products as much as possible:

Skip the sugar. Diabetes is the classical model of accelerated aging and sugar is made of empty calories anyway. The drive to consume glucose is innate, I know, but choose fresh fruit salads instead. You will get your sugar fix and some nutrients on the side.

The sweet tooth is the part most people find difficult about leading a healthy lifestyle and most traditional sweets are made of eggs, milk, butter and flour which are baked in the oven. That is the perfect recipe for advanced glycation end-products: you have proteins, sugar and high temperatures.

The result is the Maillard reaction. We already 'bake' from within as time passes by, so why add more glycation? You could try raw vegan desserts in exchange. These are made with nuts, seeds and fruits and don't involve any heating or baking, hence they are faster to make as well.

Lately, raw vegan cake shops have started to spring up everywhere. If there is no such place where you live, search online for raw vegan dessert recipes, especially if you have a weakness for sweets. Don't let a day pass without eating a salad and add as many different fresh ingredients to it as possible.

Avoid smoked meat and cheese. Same for grilled meats. In both cases you have the unhappy mix of high temperatures and proteins which easily get denatured. The consumption of these types of products is linked to digestive cancers in populations where they are consumed in high □uantity.

There are better ways to prepare animal products, so why risk it? You could try marinated fish or non-smoked fermented cheese. Eat as few animal products as possible - once per week should be enough.

Use the lowest possible temperatures when cooking. If you are baking peppers, you could use a lower temperature and a longer time than if you would bake meat. Of course, you don't want to eat raw meats and get infections. Just use your best judgment when cooking.

Use high moisture levels when cooking. It's much better to boil and broil than to roast or fry ingredients. If you are a fan of crispy food, that would be difficult to implement. On the other hand, there are many fresh vegetables and fruits that are naturally crispy if you feel the need for it - peppers anyone?

You don't need oil to cook. A ceramic pan/pot and a little bit of water will do and food will not stick. Cleaning is a breeze afterwards.

Avoid heating up fats. You can always add cheese, avocado, nuts and seeds in your recipes later on. Don't bake, fry or roast these. Cheese will melt anyway if you place it over steamy fresh potatoes and the end result will be just as delicious.

Water should be your default beverage. Everything else - soups, teas, etc - is a bonus and they will never replace water, even if the human body will work with what is available and it will extract water from them.

People get more dehydrated with age anyway and many substances precipitate if you don't drink enough water, so why speed things up when water is so freely available and cheap? I guess if you are able to read this post, then access to clean water is not an issue. Unfortunately, that's not the case for everybody.

Eat as fresh as possible. If you want to eat meat or seafood, get it fresh and only use frozen ingredients if nothing else is available. Don't cook more food than you eat in one sitting. Heated food is not as fresh or delicious as readily prepared one.

Chapter 21

7 practical recipes throughout the week

Weekly program

Monday:

Breakfast: Green tea with ginger wholemeal bread and blackberry jam

Snack: 100% blueberry juice

Lunch: Mixed vegetables seasoned with a drizzle of olive oil;

Snack: 50 grams of nuts

Dinner: anchovy pie with beetroot

Tuesday:

Breakfast: Half a cup of whole grains or oats

Snack: A seasonal fruit

Lunch: Whole curry risotto

Snack: White yogurt with live milk enzymes

Dinner: Grilled salmon on a bed of mixed vegetables seasoned with a drizzle of olive oil.

Wednesday:

Breakfast: Infusion of ginger semolina bread and currant jam

Snack: An apple

Lunch: Onion soup, rye bread and fennel bread

Snack: Two squares of dark chocolate

Dinner: Mackerel with lemon and green beans

Thursday:

Breakfast: Green tea or freshly squeezed orange juice

Snack: 6 almonds

Lunch: plenty of vegetables and a spoonful of extra virgin olive oil

Snack: 125 grams of low-fat yogurt with little pieces of fruit

Dinner: Lentil balls and lettuce side dish

Friday:

Breakfast: bread or rusks or biscuits or cereals

Snack: a seasonal fruit

Lunch: cooked or raw vegetables

Snack: fruit ice cream

Dinner: 120 grams of turkey or defatted chicken

Saturday:

Breakfast: Rusks or 1 wholemeal sandwich / rye or whole grains with jam or honey

Snack: A banana

Lunch: Spelled salad with legumes, vegetables and a side of spinach

Snack: 6 nuts

Dinner: Warm octopus, zucchini and chicory

Sunday:

Breakfast: a jar of natural soy yogurt

Snack: Pomegranate juice 100%

Lunch: 80 grams of mackerel / tuna in brine

Snack: 30 grams of hazelnuts

Dinner: 150 grams of white fish with simple cooking

Recommended to drink a glass of wine or good water.

Importantly, in addition to following an anti-inflammatory diet it is good practice to perform regular physical activity and sleep at least 8 hours.

An anti-inflammatory diet, along with regular exercise and sufficient rest can therefore bring many benefits.

Conclusion

You are what you eat' implies that certain foods can be good or bad for you. They are bad if they are inflammatory foods and good if they are not. If you are a doctor who treats inflammatory conditions, like neck pain or low back pain, wouldn't you want your patients to eat foods that help to reduce inflammation as oppose to consuming inflammatory foods?

This GUIDE begins with the premise that eating certain foods can actually make things hurt worse-increases inflammation-while eating other foods can actually help lessen pain and promote faster healing.

These are known as anti-inflammatory foods and they are closely related to competing omega fatty acids. Swelling, redness, heat and pain occur when tissue become inflamed. It may be overt, like a sprained ankle, or hidden beneath the skin, like in your stomach.

An example of inflammatory foods are those high in refined or hydrogenated vegetable oils, like potato chips and many baked goods. Refined oils and trans fats are used by manufacturers to extend the shelf life of their products.

They are notorious preservatives. On the other hand, olive oil, avocado oil and grape seed oil are natural and are known to be anti-inflammatory. Salmon is very high on the list of ant-inflammatory foods.

The reason has to do with the competing omega fatty acids. "A healthy diet contains a balance of omega-3 and omega-6 fatty acids. Omega-3 fatty acids help reduce inflammation, and some omega-6 fatty acids tend to promote inflammation

Now, red meats, such as a good, juicy steak, are high in omega-6 fatty acids. So, does that make it bad? No. It's extremely good for you. A good steak is loaded with essential amino acids and other nutrients.

It's just that the key to improving health and reducing inflammation is to balance the amount of omega-6 (e.g., nuts, eggs, poultry, cream, cheese, butter) against the omega-3 (e.g., salmon, tuna, turkey). The saturated fats contained in omega-6 foods compete with the omega-3 foods for vital digestive enzymes, like seagulls fighting over french fries on the boardwalk.

Along with omega-3's, omega-6's play a crucial role in brain function as well as normal growth and development." Anti-inflammatory foods include colorful, high fiber vegetables like sweet peppers, celery, raw carrots, onions, garlic, broccoli, cauliflower, cucumber, apples, pears, berries, nuts, grapes, bananas, citrus fruits and so on (omega-3's).

So here's my advice: Limit fatty animal products like red meats and dairy products. Instead, eat more lean cuts of chicken, turkey and fish. Olive oils and avocado can and should replace unhealthy oils from corn, soybeans, safflower, sunflower and other vegetable oils.

Sweets should be limited, including all bakery products like cookies, cakes, pies and breads. We all know that our modern diet of processed and fast foods tends to generate inflammation and other evils, like obesity. To counteract bad eating, give close consideration to the competing omega fatty acids.